THE ACID WATCHER DIET COOKBOOK

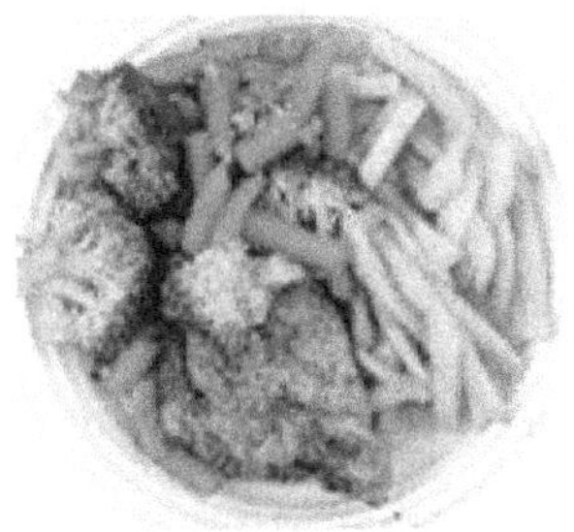

1800 Days Delicious And Nourishing Recipes to Prevent and Heal Acid Reflux Disease and Manage LPR Symptoms.

Mattie Morgan

Copyright © 2024 by Mattie Morgan

Table of Contents

INTRODUCTION

Few threads in our everyday lives weave a more complicated pattern than the decisions we make about what we eat. From the minute we wake up until the final mouthful before bedtime, our bodies react to the food we consume, impacting not just our energy levels but also our entire well-being.

For many people, the connection between nutrition and health is especially poignant when dealing with acid reflux and its more elusive cousin, Laryngopharyngeal Reflux (LPR). The Acid Watcher Diet Cookbook emerges as a culinary guide, providing not only meals but also a road map for dealing with the pain caused by these illnesses.

To begin, it is critical to understand the complexities of acid reflux and LPR. Acid reflux occurs when stomach acid regurgitates into the esophagus, causing symptoms including heartburn, chest pain, and regurgitation. LPR, on the other hand, goes beyond the esophagus to impact the neck and even the voice box.

Symptoms include a chronic cough, hoarseness, throat clearing, and a persistent sense of a lump in the throat. While both illnesses share the common thread of excessive stomach acid, LPR presents a more complex set of issues, usually necessitating a sophisticated approach to treatment.

Diet plays a critical role in the intricate interplay of variables that contribute to acid reflux. Certain foods and beverages can aggravate or alleviate symptoms, affecting the delicate balance of stomach acid production.

Recognizing this relationship, The Acid Watcher Diet Cookbook is based on the principle that what we eat has a significant impact on our digestive health. This cookbook is a valuable resource for anyone suffering from acid reflux and LPR, providing a tasty selection of meals that have been meticulously chosen to adhere to the Acid Watcher Diet principles.

The overall goal of the Acid Watcher Diet is to enable people to take control of their health through mindful eating. It was created as a unique dietary approach to address the underlying causes of acid reflux and LPR.

Unlike fad diets, The Acid Watcher Diet is based on a thorough study of the physiological mechanisms that underpin these illnesses.

The primary objective is to reduce the formation of excess stomach acid, which alleviates symptoms and promotes long-term health. Adopting a low-acid diet takes you on an exciting journey of self-discovery, teaching you how to traverse a world of culinary delights that not only tantalize the taste buds but also promote digestive harmony.

This cookbook serves as a guide on this journey, giving useful tools and delectable meals that make the Acid Watcher Diet an appealing and joyful lifestyle choice. Beyond symptom treatment, the Acid Watcher Diet seeks to promote a comprehensive approach to health. The diet promotes general well-being by prioritizing nutrient-dense, whole foods, which aids the body's desire for balance.

The recipes in The Acid Watcher Diet Cookbook are more than just a collection of ingredients; they demonstrate the concept that delicious, nourishing meals can be a cornerstone of health, acting as both preventative medicine and a source of pleasure.

As individuals embark on the Acid Watcher Diet, they embrace the opportunity to redefine their relationship with food.

It's not about deprivation but rather about making informed choices that prioritize well-being. Through the pages of this cookbook, readers will discover that the journey to relief from acid reflux can be a flavorful and satisfying adventure—one where every meal is an opportunity to nourish the body and soothe the soul.

In the following chapters, we will look at the Acid Watcher Diet's principles, including the low-acid meals that serve as the foundation and the acidic triggers to watch out for. The cookbook will reveal a treasure trove of dishes ranging from breakfast to dinner and every snack in between, all meant to delight taste buds while maintaining digestive health's delicate balance.

Let this cookbook be your guide and confidant in a world where the joy of eating is inextricably linked with the desire for relief from acid reflux and LPR.

CHAPTER 1:

Understanding Acid Reflux

Stomach acid, also known as gastric acid or hydrochloric acid, is an important part of the digestive process because it protects the body from dangerous bacteria and aids in the digestion of food. This powerful acid, produced by the gastric glands that line the stomach walls, generates an acidic environment that is required for a variety of processes.

First and foremost, stomach acid serves as a powerful barrier, protecting the body from any viruses that may be present in foods. Its acidic nature acts as a disinfectant, inhibiting the growth of dangerous bacteria, viruses, and parasites. Aside from its protective purpose, stomach acid starts the digestion of proteins. It stimulates pepsin, an enzyme that converts complex protein structures into smaller, more digestible components.

Furthermore, the stomach's acidic environment aids in the absorption of certain minerals, such as calcium and magnesium, as well as the activation of intrinsic factors, which is essential for vitamin B12 absorption in the small intestine. In summary, stomach acid is a complex player in the digestive orchestra, helping to maintain a careful balance that benefits both digestive health and immune function.

Symptoms of Acid Reflux and Laryngopharyngeal Reflux (LPR)

Heartburn (Acid Reflux): The primary symptom of acid reflux is a burning sensation or discomfort in the chest, which frequently rises to the throat. This happens when stomach acid rushes back into the esophagus.

Regurgitation: Acid reflux patients may notice sour or bitter-tasting fluid going up into their throat or mouth, indicating stomach content backflow.

Difficulty Swallowing (Dysphagia): Acid reflux can cause esophageal narrowing, which makes swallowing difficult. This could manifest as a feeling of food getting stuck in the throat.

Chronic Cough: Acid reflux and LPR are both associated with a chronic, dry cough. Even in the absence of usual respiratory issues, stomach acid irritation can trigger a cough reflex.

Hoarseness: or raspy voice is a common symptom of LPR caused by acid reflux into the vocal cords. This separates LPR from regular acid reflux since the symptoms extend beyond the esophagus.

Throat Clearing and Lump Sensation: People with LPR commonly need to clear their throats or have a persistent sense of a lump or tightness in the throat, referred to as a globus sensation.

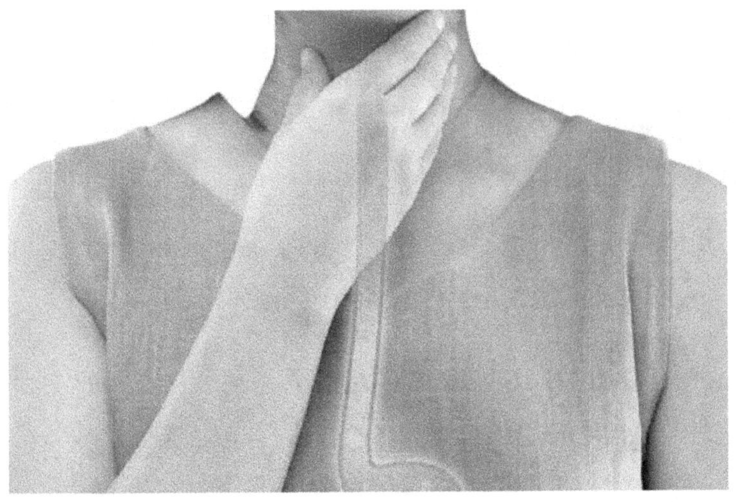

Chronic Sore Throat: Acid reflux and LPR can both cause throat irritation and inflammation, resulting in a persistent sore throat that doesn't respond to traditional throat lozenges.

Excessive Salivation: Some people may experience an increase in saliva production as their bodies try to counteract and eliminate the acidic reflux.

Understanding these symptoms is critical for a timely diagnosis and successful treatment of acid reflux and LPR, promoting relief and avoiding complications. If these symptoms persist or worsen, it is best to consult a doctor for an accurate diagnosis and personalized treatment.

Common Triggers for Acid Reflux:

Citrus Fruits: Acidic fruits such as oranges, lemons, and grapefruits can cause acid reflux by raising stomach acid and relaxing the lower esophageal sphincter (LES).

Tomatoes and Tomato-Based Products: Tomatoes are naturally acidic, and foods like tomato sauce, ketchup, and salsa can exacerbate acid reflux. The acidity may weaken the LES, allowing stomach acid to enter the esophagus.

Coffee and caffeinated beverages can relax the LES, resulting in acid reflux. Coffee, tea, and certain sodas are typical causes.

Chocolate includes both caffeine and theobromine, a chemical that can relax the LES and potentially cause acid reflux symptoms.

Spicy Foods: Hot and spicy foods can irritate the esophagus and relax the LES, causing acid reflux.

Fatty and Fried Foods: High-fat meals, such as fried foods and fatty cuts of meat, take longer to digest and may lead to increased stomach acid production, causing acid reflux.

Peppermint and Mint: While peppermint can help with indigestion, it can also relax the LES, which can cause acid reflux symptoms in some people.

Onions and garlic: These tasty additives to meals can relax the LES and increase stomach acid production, potentially causing acid reflux.

Understanding and limiting your consumption of these common triggers is critical for treating and avoiding acid reflux. While triggers differ from person to person, understanding these common causes can help individuals make smart food choices to lessen the risk of acid reflux episodes.

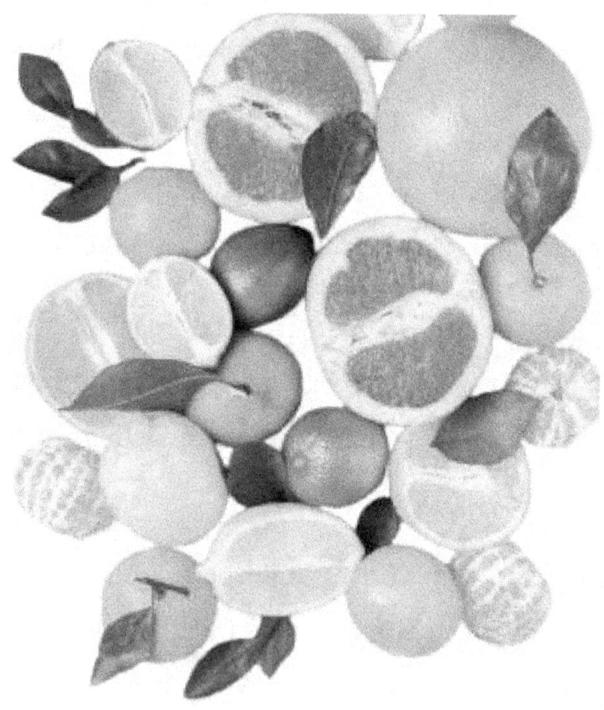

Citrus Fruits (triggers)

CHAPTER 2:

The Acid Watcher Diet Principles

The Acid Watcher Diet is based on core principles designed to alleviate acid reflux and laryngopharyngeal reflux (LPR) symptoms. The diet emphasizes a low-acid approach, promoting the consumption of alkaline-rich foods while avoiding acidic triggers. It promotes a well-balanced diet of fruits, vegetables, lean meats, and whole grains, resulting in a pH-neutral body.

Beyond nutrition adjustments, the Acid Watcher Diet emphasizes the significance of meal scheduling, portion management, and lifestyle changes. Individuals who adhere to these principles hope to balance stomach acidity, ease symptoms, and promote long-term digestive health and well-being.

Balancing pH Levels in the Body

Maintaining good health requires balancing the body's pH levels. The pH scale measures whether a material is acidic or alkaline, with 7 representing neutrality, lower numbers suggesting acidity, and higher ones indicating alkalinity.

The body's internal pH balance is tightly regulated, with different organs and systems performing best within certain pH ranges. The Acid Watcher Diet focuses on alkaline-rich meals to counterbalance the acidic effects of stomach contents, fostering a more neutral pH state.

This balance is essential for enzymatic activity, nutrient absorption, and overall cell function. Individuals who follow a pH-balancing diet want to offset the negative consequences of high acidity by creating a harmonious internal environment favorable to enhanced digestion and general well-being.

Role of Alkaline Foods and Beverages

Alkaline meals and beverages play an important function in maintaining the body's pH equilibrium. Alkaline-rich meals, such as some fruits, vegetables, and legumes, help to balance the acidity created during digestion. The Acid Watcher Diet stresses the use of alkaline foods to counteract the effects of stomach acid, lowering the risk of acid reflux and other symptoms.

Alkaline liquids, particularly water with a higher pH, help to neutralize excess acid in the stomach. By including these elements in your diet, you create an alkaline environment that promotes general health, good digestion, and relief from acid reflux and laryngopharyngeal reflux (LPR). The Acid Watcher Diet's strategy for promoting digestive harmony relies heavily on the intentional integration of alkaline foods and beverages.

Importance of Low-Acid Eating

Low-acid eating is important since it directly reduces symptoms associated with acid reflux and laryngopharyngeal reflux (LPR). The Acid Watcher Diet is based on low-acid eating to reduce stomach acid production and alleviate pain. You can reduce your risk of acid reflux by eating foods with lower acidity, such as non-citrus fruits, vegetables, and lean meats.

This dietary approach helps to prevent irritation of the esophagus and throat, lowering the risk of heartburn, regurgitation, and other symptoms. The Acid Watcher Diet acknowledges that food choices are critical in managing both disorders, and low-acid eating emerges as a crucial strategy for promoting digestive health and improving general quality of life for people suffering from acid reflux and LPR.

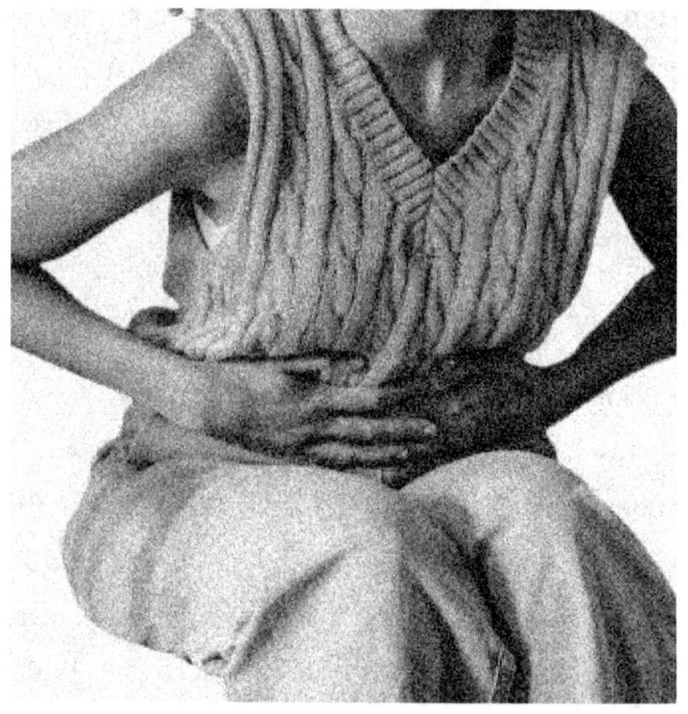

CHAPTER 3:

Low-Acid Foods

Low-acid foods are an important component of dietary treatments such as The Acid Watcher Diet, which aims to relieve symptoms of acid reflux and laryngopharyngeal reflux (LPR). These meals have a pH closer to neutral, lowering the chance of acid reflux episodes. Non-citrus fruits such as bananas and melons, vegetables like broccoli and sweet potatoes, and lean meats like poultry and fish are all good examples. Individuals who prioritize low-acid foods can establish a digestive environment that reduces stomach acid production, improving symptom alleviation and general well-being.

List of Recommended Fruits

Bananas, Melons (e.g., cantaloupe, honeydew, watermelon), Pears, Apples, Papaya, Avocado, Berries (e.g., strawberries, blueberries, raspberries), Peaches, Plums, Mango, Grapes, Cherries, Apricots, Kiwi, Pineapple, Oranges (in moderation for some; varies among individuals), Tangerines, Grapefruit (in moderation for some; varies among individuals), Cranberries, Coconut

While these fruits are generally considered low-acid, individual reactions may vary. It's advisable for individuals with acid reflux or LPR to pay attention to their own tolerance levels and make adjustments based on personal experiences.

Selection of Vegetables and Leafy Greens

Vegetables: Broccoli, Carrots, Cucumbers, Zucchini, Sweet potatoes, Cabbage, Green beans, Spinach, Kale, Celery, Asparagus, Bell peppers, Cauliflower, Potatoes (preferably sweet potatoes), Mushrooms, Brussels sprouts, Eggplant, Radishes, Butternut squash, Peas

Leafy Greens:, Lettuce (varieties such as romaine, iceberg, and butter head), Spinach, Kale, Swiss chard, Collard greens, Arugula, Watercress, Mustard greens, Bok choy, Turnip greens, Endive, Radicchio, Dandelion greens, Beet greens, Chicory.

Lean Proteins for Acid Reflux Relief

Lean proteins play a crucial role in acid reflux relief by providing essential nutrients without adding excessive fat, a common trigger for acid reflux. Opting for lean protein

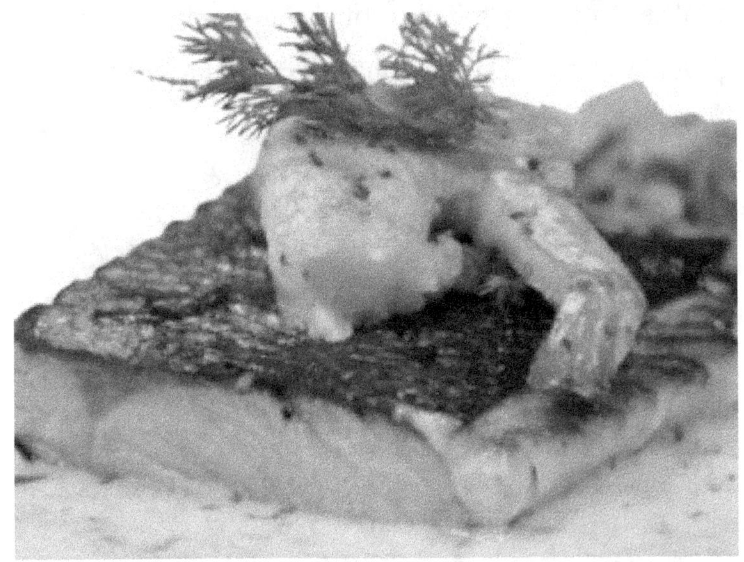

sources, such as poultry, fish, tofu, legumes, and lean cuts of meat, ensures a lower fat content in meals. High-fat foods can relax the lower esophageal sphincter (LES), allowing stomach acid to flow back into the esophagus.

In contrast, lean proteins offer a substantial source of amino acids without the added burden of excess fat, promoting better digestion and reducing the likelihood of acid reflux symptoms. The Acid Watcher Diet emphasizes the inclusion of lean proteins to provide a satisfying and nourishing foundation for meals while supporting digestive health and offering relief from the discomfort associated with acid reflux and laryngopharyngeal reflux (LPR).

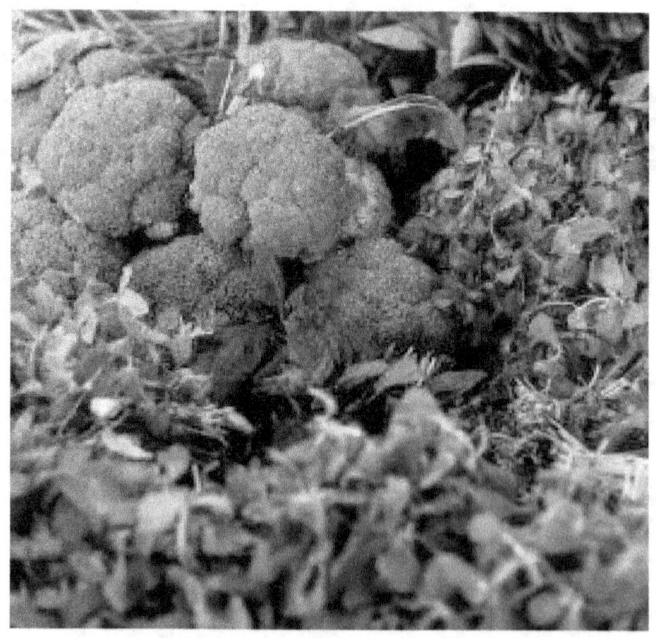

Leafy Green

CHAPTER 4:

Alkaline Water and Hydration

Alkaline water plays an important part in acid reflux control by promoting an alkaline environment within the body. With a higher pH, alkaline water is thought to neutralize excess stomach acid, potentially lowering the risk of acid reflux and laryngopharyngeal reflux (LPR) symptoms.

While scientific proof for its usefulness is limited, some people find relief from symptoms by integrating alkaline water into their daily hydration routine. Adequate hydration is important for overall health and, in the case of acid reflux, helps to dilute stomach acid. The Acid Watcher Diet supports alkaline water as part of its approach to staying hydrated and creating an internal environment that promotes digestive balance and relief from acid-related pain.

Benefits of Alkaline Water

Neutralize Stomach Acid: Some advocates believe that alkaline water, which has a higher pH, might help neutralize excess stomach acid, potentially lowering acid reflux symptoms.

Hydration: Alkaline water keeps you hydrated, which is vital for good health. Proper hydration promotes biological processes, including digestion, and helps to prevent dehydration, which can worsen acid reflux symptoms.

Antioxidant properties: Some alkaline waters claim to have antioxidant qualities, which might help battle oxidative stress. Antioxidants are thought to neutralize free radicals, which promotes cellular health.

Bone Health: According to some studies, alkaline water may improve bone health by lowering indicators of bone resorption, but more study is needed to provide definitive proof.

Detoxification: alkaline water helps the body detoxify by neutralizing acidic waste products. However, the body's natural processes, particularly the kidneys, maintain acid-base balance.

Guidelines for Proper Hydration and Limiting Acidic Beverages

Proper hydration is vital for general health and helps to manage acid reflux. The Acid Watcher Diet emphasizes hydration recommendations, including careful beverage selection. Firstly, people are advised to drink enough water throughout the day. Water is a neutral beverage that helps to dilute stomach acid, promote digestion, and prevent dehydration.

Another important consideration is to limit the use of acidic drinks. Carbonated drinks, caffeinated beverages such as coffee and tea, and citrus juices can all contribute to increased stomach acidity and cause acid reflux symptoms. The guidelines recommend limiting or avoiding acidic beverages to maintain a more alkaline environment in the body.

Furthermore, people are advised to be cautious of their beverage choices during meals. Excessive drinking while eating might dilute stomach acid, thereby impeding appropriate digestion. It is recommended to drink water between meals rather than with or shortly after them to allow for healthy digestion processes.

In following The Acid Watcher Diet, strive to maintain digestive health, reduce acid reflux symptoms, and cultivate an internal environment favorable to general well-being by sticking to these hydration rules and choosing beverages wisely.

CHAPTER 5:

Meal Timing and Portion Control

The Acid Watcher Diet emphasizes meal timing and quantity control as key factors in reducing acid reflux symptoms. The dietary guide recommends smaller, more frequent meals throughout the day, spaced out at least three hours apart.

This method avoids overloading the stomach, lowering the danger of excessive acid production and reflux. Portion control ensures that each meal is balanced and does not stress the digestive system.

Avoiding large, heavy meals close to bedtime is also recommended to ensure good digestion and reduce the risk of overnight reflux. The fundamentals of meal timing and amount management are essential for generating a digestive environment that promotes acid reflux treatment.

Eating Smaller, Frequent Meals

The Acid Watcher Diet advocates eating smaller, more frequent meals throughout the day to help with acid reflux symptoms. This method has various advantages, including limiting overeating, which can result in increased stomach acid production and reflux. Spreading meal consumption throughout the day helps to maintain a stable blood sugar level, preventing spikes and crashes that can cause acid reflux.

Smaller, more balanced meals also lessen the possibility of exerting too much pressure on the lower esophageal sphincter (LES), lowering the danger of stomach acid refluxing back into the esophagus. Ultimately, this approach creates a digestive environment that supports acid reflux relief, giving you a long-term and realistic dietary strategy for dealing with the symptoms.

Avoiding Late-Night Eating

Late-night eating is problematic for The Acid Watcher Diet since it might exacerbate acid reflux symptoms. The diet prohibits eating too close to sleep to allow for appropriate digestion before lying to rest.

When people eat late at night, gravity's ability to hold stomach contents down during sleep is weakened, raising the risk of acid reflux.

Furthermore, the body's normal nightly drop in saliva production, which is responsible for neutralizing acid, exacerbates the problem. The Acid Watcher Diet recommends avoiding late-night snacking to create an atmosphere that reduces the likelihood of reflux, supporting improved sleep quality and general digestive well-being. Those who follow these guidelines have been able to stop the pattern of nightly acid reflux and aid in their quest for relief.

Portion Control for Acid Reflux Prevention

Portion control is an essential component of acid reflux prevention. Those who moderate their portion sizes lower their risk of overloading the stomach, which can result in excess acid production and reflux. Smaller, more balanced meals are recommended to ensure proper digestion and reduce strain on the lower esophageal sphincter (LES).

The diet stresses that bigger servings may help relax the LES, allowing stomach acid to flow back into the esophagus. Portion control not only helps to avoid acid reflux, but it also helps with weight management because excess weight can lead to increased intraabdominal pressure. Those who practice portion control as a dietary habit establish a digestive environment that promotes long-term well-being while alleviating acid reflux symptoms.

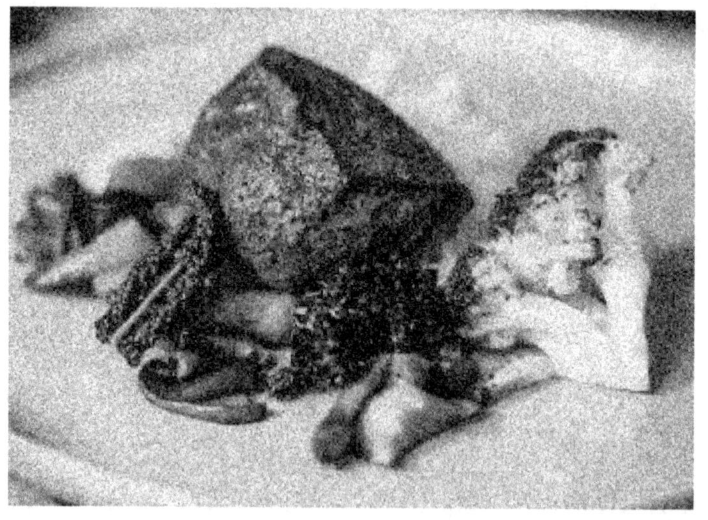

Do not forget to control you portion.

CHAPTER 8:

Acid Watcher Diet Recipes

Low-Acid Breakfasts

1. Banana and Almond Butter Smoothie

Ingredients:

- 1 ripe banana
- 1 tablespoon almond butter
- 1/2 cup Greek yogurt (non-fat or low-fat)
- 1/2 cup almond milk (unsweetened)
- 1/2 teaspoon honey (optional)
- Ice cubes

Preparation:

1. Peel and slice the banana.
2. In a blender, combine banana slices, almond butter, Greek yogurt, almond milk, and honey.
3. Blend until smooth.
4. Add ice cubes and blend again until the desired consistency is reached.

5. Pour into a glass and enjoy this creamy, low-acid smoothie.

Cooking Time: 10-15 minutes

2. Spinach and Feta Omelet

Ingredients:

- 2 large eggs
- 1 cup fresh spinach, chopped
- 2 tablespoons feta cheese, crumbled
- 1 tablespoon olive oil
- Salt and pepper to taste

Preparation:

1. In a bowl, whisk the eggs and season with salt and pepper.
2. In a nonstick skillet set over medium heat, heat the olive oil.
3. Add chopped spinach and sauté until wilted.
4. Pour the whisked eggs over the spinach.
5. Sprinkle feta cheese on top.
6. Cook until the edges set, then fold the omelet in half.

7. Continue cooking until the eggs are fully set.

8. Slide the omelet onto a plate and serve.

Cooking Time: 10-15 minutes

3. Quinoa Breakfast Bowl

Ingredients:

- 1/2 cup cooked quinoa
- 1/2 cup fresh berries (e.g., blueberries, strawberries)
- 1 tablespoon chopped nuts (e.g., almonds, walnuts)
- 1 tablespoon honey or maple syrup
- 1/2 cup Greek yogurt (non-fat or low-fat)

Preparation:

1. Cook the quinoa according to package directions and allow it to cool slightly.

2. In a bowl, layer the cooked quinoa, fresh berries, and chopped nuts.

3. Drizzle with honey or maple syrup.

4. Top with a dollop of Greek yogurt.

5. Mix together before enjoying this nutrient-packed, low-acid breakfast bowl.

Cooking Time: 10-15 minutes

4. Avocado Toast with Smoked Salmon

Ingredients:

- 1 slice whole-grain bread (low-acid)
- 1/2 ripe avocado, mashed
- 2 ounces smoked salmon
- Lemon juice (optional)
- Fresh dill for garnish
- Salt and pepper to taste

Preparation:

1. Toast the whole-grain bread slice.
2. Spread mashed avocado evenly over the toasted bread.
3. Arrange smoked salmon on top of the avocado.
4. Squeeze a little lemon juice over the salmon if desired.
5. Season with salt and pepper
6. Garnish with fresh dill.

Cooking Time: Approximately 5-7 minutes

5. Greek Yogurt Parfait

Ingredients:

- 1 cup Greek yogurt (non-fat or low-fat)
- 1/2 cup granola (low-acid)
- 1/2 cup mixed berries (e.g., raspberries, blackberries, and strawberries)
- 1 tablespoon honey

Preparation:

1. In a glass or bowl, pour the Greek yogurt, granola, and mixed berries.
2. Repeat the layers until the container is full.
3. Drizzle honey over the top.
4. Optionally, garnish with a few additional berries.

Cooking Time: No cooking required; assemble in 5 minutes.

6. Chia Seed Pudding

Ingredients:

- 2 tablespoons chia seeds
- 1/2 cup almond milk (unsweetened)
- 1/2 teaspoon vanilla extract

- 1 tablespoon maple syrup
- Fresh fruit for topping

Preparation:

1. In a bowl, combine chia seeds, almond milk, vanilla extract, and maple syrup together.
2. Stir well and refrigerate for at least 2 hours or overnight until the mixture thickens.
3. Once thickened, stir again and transfer to a serving dish.
4. Top with fresh fruit before serving.

Cooking Time: No cooking required; prep time is about 5 minutes, plus refrigeration.

7. Berry and Almond Butter Overnight Oats

Ingredients:

- 1/2 cup rolled oats
- 1/2 cup almond milk (unsweetened)
- 1 tablespoon almond butter
- 1/2 cup mixed berries (raspberries, blueberries)
- 1 teaspoon chia seeds
- 1 teaspoon honey

Preparation:

1. In a jar or container, combine rolled oats, almond milk, almond butter, mixed berries, chia seeds, and honey.
2. Stir well, ensuring the oats are fully immersed in the liquid.
3. Refrigerate overnight.
4. In the morning, give the mixture a good stir and enjoy this no-cook, low-acid breakfast.

Cooking Time: Minimal preparation time the night before

8. Sweet Potato and Spinach Breakfast Hash

Ingredients:

- 1 medium sweet potato, peeled and diced
- 1 cup fresh spinach, chopped
- 1 tablespoon olive oil
- 2 eggs
- Salt and pepper to taste

Preparation:

1. Heat the olive oil in a pan over medium heat.

2. Add diced sweet potato and sauté until tender and lightly browned.

3. Stir in chopped spinach and cook until wilted.

4. Make two wells in the hash and crack an egg into each well.

5. Cover and cook until eggs are done to your liking.

6. Season with salt and pepper before serving

Cooking Time: Approximately 15 minutes

9. Apple Cinnamon Quinoa Porridge

Ingredients:

- 1/2 cup cooked quinoa
- 1 apple, peeled and diced
- 1/2 teaspoon cinnamon
- 1 tablespoon almond butter
- 1 teaspoon honey

Preparation:

1. In a bowl, combine cooked quinoa, diced apple, cinnamon, almond butter, and honey.

2. Stir well to evenly distribute the ingredients.

3. Microwave for a minute or warm on the stove until heated through.

4. Enjoy this comforting, low-acid quinoa porridge.

Cooking Time: Approximately 5 minutes

10. Spinach and Mushroom Egg Muffins

Ingredients:

- 4 large eggs
- 1 cup fresh spinach, chopped
- 1/2 cup mushrooms, diced
- 1/4 cup feta cheese, crumbled
- 1 tablespoon olive oil
- Salt and pepper to taste

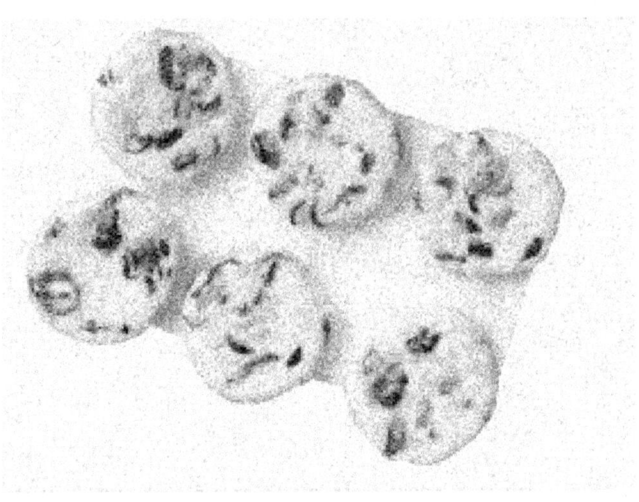

Preparation:

1. Preheat the oven to 350°F (175°C).
2. In a skillet, heat olive oil over medium heat.
3. Add diced mushrooms and sauté until softened.
4. Add chopped spinach and cook until wilted.
5. Beat the eggs in a bowl and season with salt and pepper.
6. Grease a muffin tin and distribute the mushroom and spinach mixture evenly.
7. Pour the beaten eggs over each cup.
8. Top with crumbled feta cheese.
9. Bake in the preheated oven for 15-20 minutes or until the eggs are set.
10. Allow the egg muffins to cool slightly before serving.

Cooking Time: Approximately 20 minutes

1. Grilled Chicken and Quinoa Salad

Ingredients:

- 1 cup cooked quinoa
- 6 oz grilled chicken breast, sliced
- 1 cup cherry tomatoes, halved
- 1 cucumber, diced
- 1/4 cup red onion, finely chopped
- 2 tablespoons feta cheese, crumbled
- Fresh basil, chopped
- Olive oil and balsamic vinegar for dressing
- Salt and pepper to taste

Preparation:

1. In a large bowl, combine cooked quinoa, grilled chicken slices, cherry tomatoes, cucumber, red onion, and feta cheese.
2. Sprinkle with balsamic vinegar and olive oil.
3. Add salt and pepper to taste.
4. Toss the ingredients until well combined.
5. Sprinkle fresh basil on top.

6. Serve this refreshing and nutritious salad.

Cooking Time: Grilling chicken may take around 15-20 minutes; overall assembly time is about 10 minutes

2. Lemon Herb Baked Cod

Ingredients:

- 2 cod fillets
- 1 lemon, sliced
- 2 tablespoons fresh parsley, chopped
- 1 tablespoon olive oil
- Garlic powder, salt, and pepper to taste

Preparation:

1. Preheat the oven to 375°F (190°C).
2. Put the cod fillets onto a baking sheet.
3. Drizzle olive oil over the fillets and season with garlic powder, salt, and pepper.
4. Arrange lemon slices on top and sprinkle with chopped parsley.
5. Bake in the preheated oven for 15-20 minutes or until the cod is cooked through

6. Serve with a side of steamed vegetables or a green
   salad.

Cooking Time: Approximately 20 minutes

3. Quinoa-Stuffed Bell Peppers

Ingredients:

- 4 bell peppers, halved and seeds removed
- 1 cup cooked quinoa
- 1 can (15 oz) black beans, drained and rinsed
- 1 cup corn kernels (fresh or frozen)
- 1 cup cherry tomatoes, diced
- 1/2 cup red onion, finely chopped
- 1 teaspoon ground cumin
- 1/2 teaspoon chili powder
- Salt and pepper to taste
- Shredded cheddar cheese for topping (optional)

Preparation:

1. Preheat the oven to 375°F (190°C).
2. In a bowl, mix cooked quinoa, black beans, corn,
   cherry tomatoes, red onion, cumin, chili powder,
   salt, and pepper.

3. Stuff each bell pepper half with the quinoa mixture.

4. Arrange the stuffed peppers on a baking pan.

5. If desired, top each pepper with shredded cheddar cheese.

6. Bake in the preheated oven for 25-30 minutes or until the peppers is tender.

7. Serve these flavorful quinoa-stuffed peppers for a satisfying lunch.

Cooking Time: Approximately 30 minutes

4. Turkey and Avocado Wrap

Ingredients:

- 1 whole-grain wrap
- 4 oz sliced turkey breast
- 1/2 avocado, sliced
- 1 cup mixed greens (e.g., spinach, arugula)
- 1 tablespoon Greek yogurt
- 1 teaspoon Dijon mustard
- Salt and pepper to taste

Preparation:

1. Lay out the whole-grain wrap.

2. Spread Greek yogurt and Dijon mustard on the wrap.

3. Layer sliced turkey, avocado, and mixed greens on top.

4. Season with salt and pepper.

5. Roll the wrap tightly and slice in half.

6. Secure with toothpicks if needed.

7. Enjoy this easy and nutritious turkey and avocado wrap.

Cooking Time: No cooking required; assembly time is about 5 minutes

5. Quinoa and Vegetable Stir-Fry

Ingredients:

- 1 cup cooked quinoa
- 1 cup broccoli florets
- 1 bell pepper, sliced
- 1 carrot, julienned
- 1/2 cup snap peas
- 2 tablespoons low-sodium soy sauce
- 1 tablespoon sesame oil
- 1 teaspoon grated ginger

- 1 clove garlic, minced

- Sesame seeds for garnish

Preparation:

1. In a wok or skillet, heat sesame oil over medium-high heat.
2. Add broccoli, bell pepper, carrot, and snap peas.
3. Stir-fry until vegetables are crisp-tender.
4. Add cooked quinoa to the vegetables.
5. In a small bowl, mix soy sauce, grated ginger, and minced garlic.
6. Pour the sauce over the quinoa and vegetables, toss to combine.
7. Garnish with sesame seeds before serving.

Cooking Time: Approximately 15 minutes

6. Chickpea and Spinach Salad

Ingredients:

- 1 can (15 oz) chickpeas, drained and rinsed

- 2 cups fresh spinach

- 1 cucumber, diced

- 1 cup cherry tomatoes, halved

- 1/4 cup red onion, thinly sliced

- Feta cheese for topping (optional)

- Balsamic vinaigrette dressing

- Salt and pepper to taste

Preparation:

1. In a large bowl, combine chickpeas, fresh spinach, cucumber, cherry tomatoes, and red onion.

2. Drizzle with balsamic vinaigrette dressing.

3. Season with salt and pepper.

4. Toss the salad until ingredients are well coated.

5. Top with feta cheese if desired.

6. Serve this light and flavorful chickpea and spinach salad.

Cooking Time: No cooking required; assembly time is about 10 minutes

7. Shrimp and Vegetable Stir-Fry

Ingredients:

- 1 cup shrimp, peeled and deveined

- 1 cup broccoli florets

- 1 bell pepper, thinly sliced

- 1 carrot, julienned
- 1/2 cup snow peas
- 2 tablespoons low-sodium soy sauce
- 1 tablespoon olive oil
- 1 teaspoon minced garlic
- 1 teaspoon grated ginger
- Brown rice for serving

Preparation:

1. In a wok or skillet, heat olive oil over medium-high heat.
2. Add shrimp and stir-fry until pink and opaque.
3. Add broccoli, bell pepper, carrot, and snow peas.
4. Stir-fry until vegetables are tender-crisp.
5. In a small bowl, mix soy sauce, minced garlic, and grated ginger.
6. Pour the sauce over the shrimp and vegetables, toss to coat.
7. Serve over brown rice for a satisfying and low-acid lunch.

Cooking Time: Approximately 15 minutes

8. Quinoa and Black Bean Bowl

Ingredients:

- 1 cup cooked quinoa
- 1 can (15 oz) black beans, drained and rinsed
- 1 avocado, diced
- 1/2 cup corn kernels (fresh or frozen)
- 1/4 cup red onion, finely chopped
- Fresh cilantro for garnish
- Lime wedges
- Salt and pepper to taste

Preparation:

1. In a bowl, combine cooked quinoa, black beans, diced avocado, corn, and red onion.
2. Season with salt and pepper.
3. Toss the ingredients until well combined.
4. Garnish with fresh cilantro and serve with lime wedges for squeezing.

Cooking Time: Approximately 10 minutes

9. Mediterranean Chickpea Salad

Ingredients:

- 1 can (15 oz) chickpeas, drained and rinsed
- 1 cucumber, diced
- 1 cup cherry tomatoes, halved
- 1/4 cup red onion, thinly sliced
- Kalamata olives, pitted and sliced
- Feta cheese, crumbled
- Olive oil and red wine vinegar for dressing
- Fresh oregano for garnish
- Salt and pepper to taste

Preparation:

1. In a large bowl, combine chickpeas, cucumber, cherry tomatoes, red onion, olives, and feta cheese.
2. Drizzle with both olive oil and red wine vinegar.
3. Season with salt and pepper.
4. Toss the salad until ingredients are well coated.
5. Garnish with fresh oregano.

Cooking Time: No cooking required; assembly time is about 10 minutes

10. Salmon and Quinoa Bowl

Ingredients:

- 1 cup cooked quinoa
- 6 oz baked or grilled salmon, flaked
- 1 cup steamed broccoli florets
- 1/2 avocado, sliced
- 1/4 cup cherry tomatoes, halved
- 2 tablespoons lemon juice
- 1 tablespoon olive oil
- Fresh dill for garnish
- Salt and pepper to taste

Preparation:

1. In a bowl, combine cooked quinoa, flaked salmon, steamed broccoli, avocado slices, and cherry tomatoes.
2. Drizzle with lemon juice and olive oil.
3. Add pepper and salt according to taste.
4. Toss the ingredients gently until well mixed.
5. Garnish with fresh dill before serving.

Cooking Time: Approximately 20 minutes (includes baking or grilling time for salmon).

1. Baked Lemon Herb Chicken

Ingredients:

- 4 boneless, skinless chicken breasts
- 2 lemons, juiced
- 2 tablespoons olive oil
- 2 teaspoons dried oregano
- 1 teaspoon dried thyme
- 1 teaspoon garlic powder
- Salt and pepper to taste
- Fresh parsley for garnish

Preparation:

1. Preheat the oven to 375°F (190°C).
2. In a bowl, whisk together lemon juice, olive oil, oregano, thyme, garlic powder, salt, and pepper.
3. Lay the chicken breasts in a baking dish and drizzle the lemon herb mixture over them.
4. Bake for 25-30 minutes or until the chicken is cooked through.
5. Garnish with fresh parsley before serving.

Cooking Time: Approximately 30 minutes

2. Quinoa and Vegetable Stuffed Bell Peppers

Ingredients:

- 4 bell peppers, halved and seeds removed
- 1 cup cooked quinoa
- 1 can (15 oz) black beans, drained and rinsed
- 1 cup corn kernels (fresh or frozen)
- 1 cup cherry tomatoes, diced
- 1/4 cup red onion, finely chopped
- 1 teaspoon ground cumin
- 1/2 teaspoon chili powder
- Salt and pepper to taste
- Shredded cheddar cheese for topping (optional)

Preparation:

1. Preheat the oven to 375°F (190°C).
2. In a bowl, mix cooked quinoa, black beans, corn, cherry tomatoes, red onion, cumin, chili powder, salt, and pepper.
3. Stuff each bell pepper half with the quinoa mixture.
4. Arrange the stuffed peppers on a baking pan.
5. If desired, top each pepper with shredded cheddar cheese.

6. Bake in the preheated oven for 25-30 minutes or until the peppers are tender.

7. Serve these flavorful quinoa-stuffed peppers.

Cooking Time: Approximately 30 minutes

3. Grilled Salmon with Asparagus

Ingredients:

- 4 salmon fillets
- 1 bunch asparagus, trimmed
- 2 tablespoons olive oil
- 2 cloves garlic, minced
- 1 lemon, sliced
- Fresh dill for garnish
- Salt and pepper to taste

Preparation:

1. Preheat the grill to medium-high heat.
2. In a bowl, mix olive oil, minced garlic, salt, and pepper.
3. Brush the salmon fillets and asparagus with the olive oil mixture.
4. Place the salmon fillets and asparagus on the grill.

5. Grill the salmon for about 4-5 minutes per side or until cooked through.

6. Grill the asparagus for 3-4 minutes, turning occasionally.

7. Garnish with fresh dill and lemon slices before serving.

Cooking Time: Approximately 15 minutes

4. Vegetable and Chickpea Curry

Ingredients:

- 1 can (15 oz) chickpeas, drained and rinsed
- 1 cup cauliflower florets
- 1 cup broccoli florets
- 1 carrot, sliced
- 1 bell pepper, diced
- 1 onion, finely chopped
- 2 cloves garlic, minced
- 1 can (14 oz) diced tomatoes (low-acid)
- 1 can (14 oz) unsweetened coconut milk
- 2 tablespoons curry powder
- 1 teaspoon turmeric
- 1 tablespoon olive oil

- Salt and pepper to taste
- Fresh cilantro for garnish

Preparation:

1. Heat olive oil over medium heat in a big pot.
2. Add chopped onion and garlic, sauté until softened.
3. Stir in curry powder and turmeric.
4. Add chickpeas, cauliflower, broccoli, carrot, and bell pepper.
5. Pour in diced tomatoes and coconut milk.
6. Simmer for 20-25 minutes or until vegetables are tender.
7. Season with salt and pepper.
8. Garnish with fresh cilantro before serving.
9. Serve over rice or quinoa.

Cooking Time: Approximately 30 minutes

5. Turkey and Spinach Stuffed Mushrooms

Ingredients:

- 12 large mushrooms, cleaned and stems removed
- 1/2 pound ground turkey
- 1 cup fresh spinach, chopped

- 1/4 cup onion, finely chopped
- 2 cloves garlic, minced
- 1/4 cup Parmesan cheese, grated
- 1 tablespoon olive oil
- Salt and pepper to taste

Preparation:

1. Preheat the oven to 375°F (190°C).
2. In a skillet, heat olive oil over medium heat.
3. Add chopped onion and garlic, sauté until softened.
4. Add ground turkey and cook until browned.
5. Stir in chopped spinach and cook until wilted.
6. Season with salt and pepper.
7. Spoon the turkey and spinach mixture into the mushroom caps.
8. Place stuffed mushrooms on a baking sheet and sprinkle with Parmesan cheese.
9. Bake for 15-20 minutes or until mushrooms are tender.
10. Serve these tasty stuffed mushrooms as a low-acid appetizer or main dish.

Cooking Time: Approximately 25 minutes

6. Lemon Garlic Shrimp and Zucchini Noodles

Ingredients:

- 1 pound shrimp, peeled and deveined
- 4 medium zucchinis, spiralized into noodles
- 3 tablespoons olive oil
- 3 cloves garlic, minced
- 1 lemon, juiced
- 1 teaspoon lemon zest
- Crushed red pepper flakes (optional)
- Fresh parsley for garnish
- Salt and pepper to taste

Preparation:

1. In a large skillet, heat olive oil over medium heat.
2. Add minced garlic and sauté until fragrant.
3. Add shrimp and cook until pink and opaque.
4. Toss in spiralized zucchini noodles.
5. Drizzle with lemon juice and sprinkle lemon zest.
6. Season with salt, pepper, and red pepper flakes if desired.
7. Cook for 3-5 minutes until zucchini noodles are just tender.

8. Garnish with fresh parsley before serving.

Cooking Time: Approximately 15 minutes

7. Mediterranean Baked Chicken

Ingredients:

- 4 boneless, skinless chicken breasts
- 1 cup cherry tomatoes, halved
- 1/2 cup Kalamata olives, pitted and sliced
- 1/4 cup red onion, thinly sliced
- 2 cloves garlic, minced
- 1 teaspoon dried oregano
- 1 teaspoon dried thyme
- 1/4 cup feta cheese, crumbled
- 2 tablespoons olive oil
- Salt and pepper to taste
- Fresh parsley for garnish

Preparation:

1. Preheat the oven to 375°F (190°C).
2. In a bowl, mix cherry tomatoes, olives, red onion, minced garlic, oregano, thyme, feta cheese, olive oil, salt, and pepper.

3. Place chicken breasts in a baking dish and top with the tomato mixture.

4. Bake for 25-30 minutes or until the chicken is cooked through.

5. Garnish with fresh parsley before serving.

Cooking Time: Approximately 30 minutes

8. Quinoa and Black Bean Stuffed Acorn Squash

Ingredients:

- 2 acorn squash, halved and seeds removed
- 1 cup cooked quinoa
- 1 can (15 oz) black beans, drained and rinsed
- 1 cup corn kernels (fresh or frozen)
- 1/2 cup red onion, finely chopped
- 1 teaspoon ground cumin
- 1/2 teaspoon chili powder
- Salt and pepper to taste
- Fresh cilantro for garnish

Preparation:

1. Preheat the oven to 375°F (190°C).

2. Place acorn squash halves on a baking sheet, cut side up.

3. In a bowl, mix cooked quinoa, black beans, corn, red onion, cumin, chili powder, salt, and pepper.

4. Stuff each acorn squash half with the quinoa mixture.

5. Bake in the preheated oven for 25-30 minutes or until squash is tender.

6. Garnish with fresh cilantro before serving.

Cooking Time: Approximately 30 minutes

9. Lemon Garlic Herb Tilapia

Ingredients:

- 4 tilapia fillets
- 2 lemons, juiced
- 3 cloves garlic, minced
- 2 tablespoons fresh parsley, chopped
- 1 tablespoon olive oil
- Salt and pepper to taste
- Lemon slices for garnish

Preparation:

1. Preheat the oven to 375°F (190°C).

2. In a bowl, whisk together lemon juice, minced garlic, chopped parsley, olive oil, salt, and pepper.

3. Place tilapia fillets in a baking dish and pour the lemon herb mixture over them.

4. Bake for 15-20 minutes or until the tilapia is cooked through.

5. Garnish with lemon slices before serving.

Cooking Time: Approximately 20 minutes

10. Greek Chicken Souvlaki Skewers

Ingredients:

- 1 pound chicken breast, cut into chunks
- 1 lemon, juiced
- 2 tablespoons olive oil
- 2 teaspoons dried oregano
- 2 cloves garlic, minced
- Salt and pepper to taste
- Tzatziki sauce for serving
- Cherry tomatoes and cucumber slices for skewering

Preparation:

1. In a bowl, mix lemon juice, olive oil, dried oregano, minced garlic, salt, and pepper.

2. Marinate chicken chunks in the mixture for at least 30 minutes.

3. Thread marinated chicken, cherry tomatoes, and cucumber slices onto skewers.

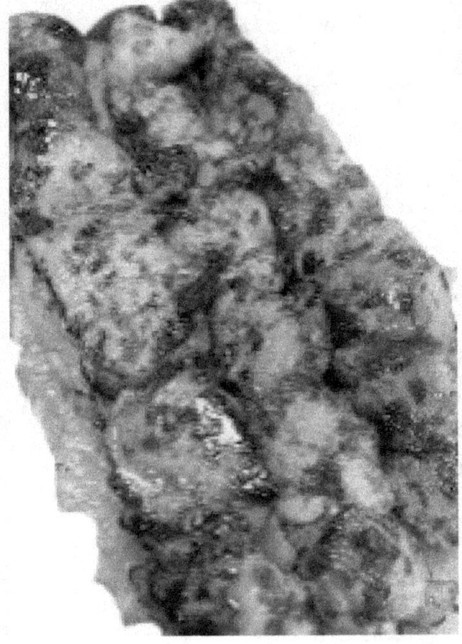

4. Grill skewers for 10-15 minutes or until chicken is cooked through.

5. Serve with a side of tzatziki sauce.

Cooking Time: Approximately 15 minutes (plus time to marinate)

1. Cucumber and Hummus Bites

Ingredients:

- 1 cucumber, sliced into rounds
- 1/2 cup hummus (low-acid)
- Cherry tomatoes, sliced (optional)
- Fresh dill for garnish
- Salt and pepper to taste

Preparation:

1. Arrange cucumber rounds on a serving platter.
2. Spoon a small amount of hummus onto each cucumber round.
3. If desired, top with a slice of cherry tomato.
4. Season with salt and pepper.
5. Garnish with fresh dill.
6. Serve these refreshing cucumber and hummus bites.

Preparation Time: Approximately 10 minutes.

2. Almond Butter and Banana Rice Cakes

Ingredients:

- Brown rice cakes
- Almond butter (low-acid)
- 1 banana, sliced
- Chia seeds for sprinkling (optional)
- Honey for drizzling (optional)

Preparation:

1. Spread almond butter on brown rice cakes.
2. Top each rice cake with banana slices.
3. Sprinkle chia seeds for added texture (optional).
4. Drizzle honey over the top if desired.
5. Enjoy these satisfying and nutritious almond butter and banana rice cakes.

Preparation Time: Approximately 5 minutes.

3. Roasted Chickpeas

Ingredients:

- 1 can (15 oz) chickpeas, drained and rinsed
- 1 tablespoon olive oil
- 1 teaspoon ground cumin

- 1/2 teaspoon smoked paprika
- Salt and pepper to taste

Preparation:

1. Preheat the oven to 400°F (200°C).
2. Pat dry chickpeas with a paper towel to remove excess moisture.
3. In a bowl, toss chickpeas with olive oil, cumin, smoked paprika, salt, and pepper.
4. Spread chickpeas on a baking sheet in a single layer.
5. Roast in a preheated oven for 20-25 minutes, until crispy.
6. Allow to cool before serving these crunchy roasted chickpeas.

Cooking Time: Approximately 25 minutes

4. Veggie Sticks with Tzatziki

Ingredients:

- Carrot sticks
- Cucumber sticks
- Bell pepper strips
- Cherry tomatoes
- Tzatziki sauce (low-acid)

Preparation:

1. Arrange carrot sticks, cucumber sticks, bell pepper strips, and cherry tomatoes on a serving platter.
2. Serve with a side of tzatziki sauce for dipping.
3. Enjoy this fresh and crunchy veggie snack with a flavorful dip.

Preparation Time: Approximately 10 minutes.

5. Quinoa and Vegetable Sushi Rolls

Ingredients:

- Nori sheets
- 1 cup cooked quinoa
- Carrot, julienned
- Cucumber, julienned
- Avocado, sliced
- Bell pepper strips (red or yellow)
- Low-sodium soy sauce for dipping
- Pickled ginger for serving (optional)
- Wasabi for serving (optional)

Preparation:

1. Lay a nori sheet on a bamboo sushi rolling mat.
2. Spread a thin layer of cooked quinoa evenly over the nori, leaving a small border at the top.

3. Arrange julienned carrot, cucumber, avocado, and bell pepper strips along the bottom edge of the nori.
4. Carefully lift the bamboo mat and start rolling the nori and fillings away from you, using gentle pressure to shape it into a roll.
5. Seal the edge of the nori with a little water to secure the roll.
6. Repeat the process to make additional rolls.
7. Using a sharp knife, slice each roll into bite-sized pieces.
8. Serve the quinoa and vegetable sushi rolls with low-sodium soy sauce, pickled ginger, and wasabi.

Preparation Time: Approximately 20 minutes.

Dessert Alternatives

1. Grilled Peaches with Honey and Almonds

Ingredients:

- 4 ripe peaches, halved and pitted
- 2 tablespoons honey
- 1/4 cup sliced almonds
- Greek yogurt or coconut milk ice cream (optional)

Preparation:

1. Preheat the grill to medium-high heat.

2. Grill peach halves, cut side down, for 3-4 minutes or until grill marks appear.

3. Flip the peaches and grill for an additional 2-3 minutes.

4. Drizzle honey over the grilled peaches.

5. Sprinkle sliced almonds on top.

6. Serve the grilled peaches with a scoop of Greek yogurt or coconut milk ice cream if desired.

7. Enjoy this simple and delicious grilled peaches dessert.

Cooking Time: Approximately 10 minutes

2. Almond Flour Lemon Poppy Seed Muffins

Ingredients:

- 2 cups almond flour
- 1/4 cup coconut flour
- 1/2 teaspoon baking soda
- 1/4 teaspoon salt
- 3 large eggs
- 1/4 cup coconut oil, melted

- 1/4 cup honey or maple syrup
- Zest and juice of 2 lemons
- 1 tablespoon poppy seeds

Preparation:

1. Preheat the oven to 350°F/175°C and line a muffin tray with paper liners.
2. Pour almond flour, coconut flour, baking soda, and salt in a bowl and whisk together.
3. In another bowl, beat eggs and mix in melted coconut oil, honey or maple syrup, lemon zest, lemon juice, and poppy seeds.
4. Combine the wet and dry ingredients, mixing until well combined.
5. Spoon the batter into the muffin tin, filling each cup about 3/4 full.
6. Bake for eighteen-twenty minutes or until a toothpick inserted into the center comes out clean.
7. Allow the muffins to cool before serving these tasty almond flour lemon poppy seed muffins.

Cooking Time: Approximately 20 minutes

3. *Coconut Chia Pudding with Mango*

Ingredients:

- 1/4 cup chia seeds
- 1 cup coconut milk (unsweetened)
- 1 tablespoon maple syrup or honey
- 1/2 teaspoon vanilla extract
- 1 ripe mango, diced
- Shredded coconut for garnish

Preparation:

1. In a bowl, mix chia seeds, coconut milk, maple syrup or honey, and vanilla extract.
2. Stir well and refrigerate for at least 2 hours or overnight to allow the chia seeds to absorb the liquid.
3. Once the chia pudding has thickened, layer it in serving glasses with diced mango.
4. Top with shredded coconut for garnish.
5. Serve this refreshing coconut chia pudding with mango.

Preparation Time: Approximately 2 hours (including chilling time).

4. Dark Chocolate Covered Strawberries

Ingredients:

- Fresh strawberries, washed and dried
- Dark chocolate (70% cocoa or higher)
- Chopped nuts (e.g., almonds, pistachios) for coating

Preparation:

1. Melt dark chocolate in a heatproof bowl over a pot of simmering water or in the microwave.
2. Dip each strawberry into the melted chocolate, coating it halfway.
3. Roll the chocolate-covered part of the strawberry in chopped nuts.
4. Place the dipped strawberries on a parchment-lined tray.
5. Allow the chocolate to set in the refrigerator for about 30 minutes.
6. Enjoy these indulgent dark chocolate-covered strawberries as a sweet treat.

Preparation Time: Approximately 30 minutes (including setting time).

5. Apple Cinnamon Baked Oatmeal Cups

Ingredients:

- 2 cups old-fashioned oats
- 1 teaspoon baking powder
- 1/2 teaspoon cinnamon
- 1/4 teaspoon salt
- 2 ripe bananas, mashed
- 1 cup unsweetened applesauce
- 1/2 cup almond milk
- 1 teaspoon vanilla extract
- 1 apple, peeled and diced
- Chopped nuts (e.g., walnuts or almonds) for topping

Preparation:

1. Preheat the oven to 350°F/175°C and line a muffin tray with paper liners.
2. In a bowl, combine oats, baking powder, cinnamon, and salt.
3. In another bowl, mash bananas and mix in applesauce, almond milk, and vanilla extract.
4. Combine the wet and dry ingredients, and then fold in the diced apple.
5. Spoon the mixture into the muffin tin, filling each cup.
6. Top each cup with chopped nuts.
7. Bake for 25-30 minutes, or until the tops turns golden brown.

8. Allow the oatmeal cups to cool before serving.

Cooking Time: Approximately 30 minutes

6. Baked Pears with Cinnamon and Walnuts

Ingredients:

- 4 ripe but firm pears, halved and cored
- 2 tablespoons melted coconut oil
- 2 tablespoons maple syrup
- 1 teaspoon ground cinnamon
- 1/4 cup chopped walnuts

Preparation:

1. Preheat the oven to 375°F (190°C) and place pear halves in a baking dish.
2. In a small bowl, mix melted coconut oil, maple syrup, and ground cinnamon.
3. Brush the pear halves with the cinnamon mixture.
4. Sprinkle chopped walnuts over the pears.
5. Bake for 25-30 minutes or until the pears are tender.
6. Serve the baked pears with a drizzle of any remaining cinnamon mixture.

Cooking Time: Approximately 30 minutes

CONCLUSION

In conclusion, The Acid Watcher Diet Cookbook is a valuable addition to the Acid Watcher Diet, providing an array of foods that adhere to the concepts of acid reflux management and general digestive health. Throughout this cookbook, the emphasis has been on creating meals that are both delicious and low in acidity, recognizing the importance of nutrition in illnesses such as acid reflux and laryngopharyngeal reflux (LPR).

The Acid Watcher Diet Principles, as outlined and shown in this cookbook, highlight the significance of adding alkaline-rich foods, lean meats, and low-acid options to everyday meals. You can manage acid-related diseases and contribute to general well-being by concentrating on nutrient-dense meals such as fruits, vegetables, and whole grains while avoiding triggers such as acidic, spicy, or fatty foods.

The connection between diet and acid reflux is clear in each recipe's meticulous choice of ingredients and taste combination. People who have followed the principles found in this Acid Watcher Diet find relief from symptoms, avoid acid-related damage, and enjoy a healthy digestive system.

This cookbook promotes long-term health and wellness, goes beyond just a compilation of recipes, and becomes a guide to sustainable eating habits. The emphasis on whole, unprocessed foods, balanced meals, and mindful eating promotes a comprehensive approach to health. The principles provided urge people to not just manage the symptoms but also to live a lifestyle that supports digestive health, which leads to better overall health.

As you begin your journey with The Acid Watcher Diet Cookbook, it is critical to see it as a tool for empowerment, providing the ability to take charge of one's health through attentive and purposeful dietary decisions. Those who incorporate these principles into their everyday lives pave the way for long-term well-being and keep their digestive systems in balance. The Acid Watcher Diet Cookbook is a complete resource for anyone seeking long-term health, offering not just meals but also a pathway to a better, more vibrant life.

Thank you for exploring this Acid Watcher Diet Cookbook. May these recipes bring you joy and contribute to your journey towards optimal health and digestive wellness. Gratefully, Mattie Morgan.

Bonus: Weekly Meal Planner

SEVEN DAY MEAL
PLANNER

WEEK ______________

Monday

Tuesday

Wednesday

Thursday

Friday

Saturday

Sunday

To Do List

- ☐ ____________________
- ☐ ____________________
- ☐ ____________________
- ☐ ____________________
- ☐ ____________________
- ☐ ____________________
- ☐ ____________________
- ☐ ____________________
- ☐ ____________________
- ☐ ____________________
- ☐ ____________________
- ☐ ____________________

Notes

____
____
____
____
____
____
____
____

SEVEN DAY MEAL PLANNER

WEEK _________

Monday

Tuesday

Wednesday

Thursday

Friday

Saturday

Sunday

To Do List

- ☐ __________________
- ☐ __________________
- ☐ __________________
- ☐ __________________
- ☐ __________________
- ☐ __________________
- ☐ __________________
- ☐ __________________
- ☐ __________________
- ☐ __________________
- ☐ __________________
- ☐ __________________

Notes

SEVEN DAY MEAL PLANNER

WEEK _______________

Monday

Tuesday

Wednesday

Thursday

Friday

Saturday

Sunday

To Do List

- ☐ _______________
- ☐ _______________
- ☐ _______________
- ☐ _______________
- ☐ _______________
- ☐ _______________
- ☐ _______________
- ☐ _______________
- ☐ _______________
- ☐ _______________
- ☐ _______________
- ☐ _______________

Notes

____

____

____

____

____

____

____

____

____

____

SEVEN DAY MEAL PLANNER

WEEK _____________

| Monday |
| Tuesday |
| Wednesday |
| Thursday |
| Friday |
| Saturday |
| Sunday |

To Do List

- ☐ _______________
- ☐ _______________
- ☐ _______________
- ☐ _______________
- ☐ _______________
- ☐ _______________
- ☐ _______________
- ☐ _______________
- ☐ _______________
- ☐ _______________
- ☐ _______________
- ☐ _______________

Notes

____

SEVEN DAY MEAL PLANNER

WEEK _____________

Monday
Tuesday
Wednesday
Thursday
Friday
Saturday
Sunday

To Do List

- ☐ ________________
- ☐ ________________
- ☐ ________________
- ☐ ________________
- ☐ ________________
- ☐ ________________
- ☐ ________________
- ☐ ________________
- ☐ ________________
- ☐ ________________
- ☐ ________________
- ☐ ________________

Notes

SEVEN DAY MEAL PLANNER

WEEK ___________

Monday

Tuesday

Wednesday

Thursday

Friday

Saturday

Sunday

To Do List

- ☐ __________
- ☐ __________
- ☐ __________
- ☐ __________
- ☐ __________
- ☐ __________
- ☐ __________
- ☐ __________
- ☐ __________
- ☐ __________
- ☐ __________
- ☐ __________

Notes

SEVEN DAY MEAL PLANNER

WEEK _____________

Monday	**To Do List**
Tuesday	☐ _______________
Wednesday	☐ _______________
Thursday	☐ _______________
Friday	☐ _______________
Saturday	**Notes**
Sunday	

SEVEN DAY MEAL PLANNER

WEEK __________

Monday	**To Do List**
Tuesday	☐ __________
Wednesday	☐ __________
Thursday	☐ __________
Friday	☐ __________
Saturday	☐ __________
Sunday	**Notes**

SEVEN DAY MEAL PLANNER

WEEK __________

Monday

Tuesday

Wednesday

Thursday

Friday

Saturday

Sunday

To Do List

- ☐ ________________
- ☐ ________________
- ☐ ________________
- ☐ ________________
- ☐ ________________
- ☐ ________________
- ☐ ________________
- ☐ ________________
- ☐ ________________
- ☐ ________________
- ☐ ________________
- ☐ ________________

Notes

____

____

____

____

____

____

____

SEVEN DAY MEAL PLANNER

WEEK ___________

Monday

Tuesday

Wednesday

Thursday

Friday

Saturday

Sunday

To Do List

☐ ____________________
☐ ____________________
☐ ____________________
☐ ____________________
☐ ____________________
☐ ____________________
☐ ____________________
☐ ____________________
☐ ____________________
☐ ____________________
☐ ____________________

Notes

____
____
____
____
____
____
____
____
____
____